Practical Management of POTS and Related Dysautonomias

A Field Guide for Resource-Limited Clinical Care

Elizabeth Clark, MSN, CRNP

This guide is intended for educational purposes for healthcare professionals.

ISBN: (Paperback) 979-8-9951843-0-0

ISBN: (eBook) 979-8-9951843-1-7

First Edition

Language: English

Library of Congress Control Number: Pending

Published in the United States of America

Dedicated to patients who were told nothing was wrong, and to the clinicians who kept trying anyway.

Contents

How to Use This Guide

This field guide is designed for clinicians who encounter patients with orthostatic intolerance and dysautonomia in real-world clinical settings.

The goal is practical pattern recognition and symptom-guided management rather than rigid diagnostic categorization.

Many patients with dysautonomia do not fit cleanly into one subtype. Hypovolemic, neuropathic, and hyperadrenergic features frequently overlap.

Clinicians should prioritize identifying dominant symptom patterns and implementing targeted interventions.

Treatment recommendations focus on practical strategies that can be implemented in general clinical environments, including settings where specialty autonomic testing is unavailable.

Abbreviations and Key Terms

POTS – Postural Orthostatic Tachycardia Syndrome

IST – Inappropriate Sinus Tachycardia

OI – Orthostatic Intolerance

NMH – Neurally Mediated Hypotension

NOH — Neurogenic Orthostatic Hypotension

VVS — Vasovagal Syncope

MSA — Multiple System Atrophy

PAF — Pure Autonomic Failure

MCAS – Mast Cell Activation Syndrome

EDS – Ehlers–Danlos Syndrome

SFN – Small Fiber Neuropathy

ME/CFS — Myalgic Encephalomyelitis / Chronic Fatigue Syndrome

LDN – Low-Dose Naltrexone

IVIG – Intravenous Immunoglobulin

SE — Side Effect

HR – Heart Rate

BP – Blood Pressure

SBP – Systolic Blood Pressure

DBP – Diastolic Blood Pressure

PP – Pulse Pressure

OSA – Obstructive Sleep Apnea

GI – Gastrointestinal

GU - Genitourinary

TTT — Tilt Table Test

QAT — Quantitative Autonomic Testing

HRDB — Heart Rate Response to Deep Breathing

QSART — Quantitative Sudomotor Axon Reflex Test

Preface

Dysautonomia remains widely underrecognized despite the large number of patients affected. Many individuals experience years of symptoms before receiving appropriate evaluation.

Patients frequently report that their symptoms were dismissed after routine testing appeared normal.

This guide was developed to provide clinicians with a practical framework for recognizing and managing common dysautonomia presentations using tools available in everyday clinical practice.

The intent is not to replace specialty evaluation but to help clinicians recognize patterns and initiate supportive treatment when appropriate.

Disclaimer

The information contained in this guide is intended for educational purposes for licensed healthcare professionals.

This publication reflects the clinical experience and practice patterns of the author and is not intended to establish a universal standard of care. Clinical judgment should guide patient management, and treatment decisions should be individualized based on patient presentation and current medical evidence.

Medicine is an evolving field. While efforts have been made to ensure accuracy at the time of publication, new research and clinical findings may alter recommended approaches.

The author assumes no responsibility for any injury or damage resulting from the application of information contained in this guide.

About the Author

Elizabeth Clark, MSN, CRNP is a board-certified nurse practitioner with extensive clinical experience in the evaluation and management of dysautonomia and related conditions.

Her work focuses on practical approaches to improving patient function and quality of life in individuals with orthostatic intolerance and autonomic dysfunction.

Recognizing the Pattern

Postural Orthostatic Tachycardia Syndrome (POTS) and related dysautonomias often present with symptoms that appear unrelated at first glance.

Patients may report fatigue, dizziness, tachycardia, gastrointestinal symptoms, cognitive impairment, temperature dysregulation, and exercise intolerance.

Symptoms frequently worsen with upright posture and improve when lying down.

Clinicians should focus on identifying patterns rather than evaluating each symptom in isolation.

Common symptom clusters include:

• Orthostatic intolerance

• Tachycardia or palpitations

• Fatigue and post-exertional worsening

• Cognitive dysfunction ("brain fog")

• Temperature dysregulation

• Gastrointestinal symptoms

• Sleep disturbances

• Blood pooling in extremities

Evaluating Orthostatic Intolerance

Orthostatic intolerance refers to symptoms that occur in the upright position and improve with recumbency.

Patients may describe symptoms as dizziness, lightheadedness, fatigue, weakness, nausea, palpitations, or visual disturbances when standing.

A useful clinical pearl:

If symptoms improve rapidly when lying down, orthostatic intolerance should be strongly considered.

If symptoms persist when supine or are triggered by head movement while lying down, vestibular causes should also be considered.

10-Minute Stand Test

When tilt table testing is unavailable, the 10-minute stand test provides a useful clinical alternative.

Preparation

The patient should rest supine for approximately 5–10 minutes prior to testing.

Ideally testing should occur before significant fluid or sodium intake and before medications that affect heart rate or blood pressure.

Procedure

Measure heart rate and blood pressure after resting supine.

The patient then stands upright without walking.

Record heart rate and blood pressure and symptoms at:

1 minute

3 minutes

5 minutes

10 minutes

Safety Considerations

Because syncope may occur, testing should be performed with appropriate precautions.

Recommended safety measures include staff trained in CPR/BLS and access to emergency assistance if needed.

10 Minute Stand Test Interpretation

Pattern	Heart Rate Response	Blood Pressure Response	Typical Symptoms	Clinical Notes
Normal Response	HR increase <30 bpm	BP stable	Minimal symptoms	Normal physiologic response
POTS	HR increase ≥30 bpm within 10 min (or HR ≥120 bpm)	BP stable or mildly reduced	Lightheadedness, fatigue, palpitations	Chronic orthostatic intolerance with tachycardia
Hyperadrenergic POTS	HR increase ≥30 bpm	Diastolic BP rise ≥10 mmHg tremor, anxiety, adrenaline surges Often high standing norepinephrine	Tremor, anxiety, adrenaline surges	Often high standing norepinephrine (Limited confirmatory testing available)

Inappropriate Sinus Tachycardia (IST)	Elevated resting HR (>90–100) with exaggerated rise	BP usually stable	Persistent tachycardia, palpitations	Tachycardia even at rest
Orthostatic Intolerance (OI) / NMH / Reflex Hypotension	HR may increase, be labile or remain unchanged	SBP drop ≥20 mmHg or DBP drop ≥10 mmHg. May have delayed BP drop or narrowing pulse pressure	Fatigue, presyncope, orthostatic symptoms without sustained tachycardia	Delayed BP drop or narrowing pulse pressure
Vasovagal Syncope (VVS)	HR may initially increase then drop	BP drop with syncope	Dizziness, syncope, orthostatic symptoms without sustained tachycardia	Episodic reflex syncope often triggered by emotional stress, baring down, phobias or pain.

Neurogenic Orthostatic Hypotension (NOH)	HR rise minimal (<15 bpm)	Supine HTN AND BP drop ≥20/10 mmHg	Dizziness, syncope. Evaluate for neurologic features: parkinsonism, gait instability, sexual, or GI/GU dysfunction	Suggests autonomic failure; Refer to neurology or autonomic specialist

Clinical Notes

Orthostatic intolerance (OI), neurally mediated and hypotension (NMH) represent overlapping physiologic patterns and may coexist with POTS.

Many patients demonstrate mixed autonomic responses, and interpretation should consider the overall symptom pattern rather than relying on strict numerical thresholds alone.

Morning Blood Pressure Assessment Tool

Morning symptoms in dysautonomia frequently relate to overnight fluid shifts and relative hypovolemia.

Blood pressure measurements obtained before getting out of bed may provide useful clinical information.

Suggested measurements include:

• supine blood pressure upon waking

• sitting blood pressure

• standing blood pressure at 1, 3, and 5 minutes (when home standing test is indicated, e.g. flares, symptom/med changes, etc)

Morning systolic blood pressure below approximately 100 mmHg may correlate with nausea, fatigue, and difficulty initiating activity.

More severe symptoms such as retching may occur when systolic blood pressure falls below approximately 90 mmHg.

These observations should be interpreted in the context of the patient's overall clinical picture.

Morning Blood Pressure Interpretation

Morning Finding	Possible Interpretation
SBP <100 mmHg on waking	Common in hypovolemic dysautonomia; may correlate with morning nausea, fatigue, and difficulty initiating activity
SBP <90 mmHg with retching or dry heaving	Often reflects significant morning hypovolemia
Narrow pulse pressure (high DBP with lower SBP)	May suggest vascular tone dysregulation or sympathetic activation
Morning symptoms improve after sodium or fluids	Supports volume depletion as contributing factor
Standing HR increases markedly after rising	Suggests orthostatic intolerance
Symptoms improve after taking morning medication before rising	Supports pre-emptive treatment strategy

Clinical Notes

Many dysautonomia patients report difficulty waking up and initiating activity in the morning.

Some clinicians recommend taking medications such as midodrine or heart rate controlling medications immediately upon waking, while still in bed, so that pharmacologic effects begin before the patient stands.

This approach may reduce early-morning symptom burden.

Additional Observation

Morning worsening of symptoms may reflect:

• overnight diuresis

• relative hypovolemia

• autonomic instability during sleep

In selected patients, clinicians may consider strategies such as bedtime sodium intake or desmopressin to reduce overnight fluid loss.

Clinical Algorithm

Initial Clinical Suspicion:

Patient presents with symptoms such as:

• lightheadedness or dizziness

• tachycardia or palpitations

• fatigue or exercise intolerance

• brain fog or cognitive slowing

• nausea or early satiety

• temperature dysregulation

• blood pooling in extremities

Symptoms worsen when upright and improve when supine.

Step 1 — Basic Evaluation

Obtain:

• orthostatic vital signs or 10-minute stand test

• medication review

• screening labs if clinically indicated (CBC, CMP, TSH, ferritin)

Evaluate for reversible contributors such as:

- dehydration

- anemias and nutritional deficiencies

- thyroid dysfunction

- medication effects

Step 2 — Identify Dominant Physiologic Pattern

Many patients demonstrate mixed features, which may evolve over time, thus a more successful treatment for dysautonomia may be better guided by the dominant symptom pattern rather than strict diagnostic subtype.

Hypovolemic pattern:

- low or low-normal blood pressure

- morning worsening of symptoms

- improvement with salt and fluids

Hyperadrenergic pattern:

- elevated standing heart rate

- elevated diastolic blood pressure

- tremor (perceived or assessed), anxiety, or adrenaline surges|

Neuropathic pattern:

- blood pooling in extremities

• dependent discoloration

• temperature dysregulation

Step 3 — Symptom-Guided Treatment Approach

Although these conservative measures are important, they rarely resolve symptoms on their own but may enhance the effectiveness of medications.

Foundational Management

Many patients benefit from interventions aimed at improving circulating blood volume:

 increased fluid intake

• increased sodium intake

• compression garments (especially abdominal)

• recumbent or graded exercise conditioning

Traditionally Fludrocortisone (or alternatively licorice root) was the first line treatment, but it took time to know if it was beneficial, which could further frustrate dysautonomia sufferers, and risked further mental distress.

Consider faster acting options like midodrine or droxidopa in these cases, especially if the patient is already oral volume compliant.

Orthostatic symptoms / vascular tone:

→ midodrine

→ droxidopa

Low blood pressure / hypovolemia:

→ fludrocortisone

→ desmopressin

Tachycardia:

→ beta blockers

→ ivabradine (best for tachycardia induced syncope, orthostasis, low-normal BP, those receiving allergy shots, those who must carry Epi-Pens, MCAS-like subtypes, and those undergoing certain endocrine testing when results would be affected by beta-blockers.)

Fatigue / cognitive dysfunction:

→ stimulants or modafinil (select patients)

→ low dose naltrexone

→ Pyridostigmine

Neuropathic pain or autonomic modulation:

→ low dose naltrexone

→ TCAs or SNRIs in select cases

Generalized muscle weakness and/or slow gastric motility/constipation

→Pyridostigmine

Step 5 — Reassess Response

Evaluate:

• symptom improvement

• orthostatic vitals

• medication tolerance

Adjust therapy gradually.

Referral to autonomic specialists may be appropriate for complex cases.

SYMPTOM → MEDICATION TABLE

Symptom Pattern	Common Options
Low blood pressure, morning nausea	fluids, sodium, fludrocortisone, desmopressin
Orthostatic lightheadedness	midodrine, droxidopa
Tachycardia	beta blockers, ivabradine
Fatigue / brain fog	midodrine, droxidopa, pyridostigmine, stimulants, modafinil
Generalized perceived muscle weakness	pyridostigmine (refer to Neuro for identified deficit)
Neuropathic pain / central sensitization	low-dose naltrexone
Sleep disturbance / hyperadrenergic state	clonidine, guanfacine
Mast-cell symptoms	H1 blockers, H2 blockers, cromolyn
GI dysmotility	Pyridostigmine, pro-motility strategies, refer to Neuro-GI, if available

Pocket Clinical Pearls

Postural symptoms matter:

If dizziness or fatigue improves rapidly when lying down, orthostatic intolerance should be strongly considered.

Rest to digest:

Many dysautonomia patients tolerate meals better after resting supine for several minutes before eating.

Rapid IV bolus works better:

Rapid administration of normal saline (500–1000 mL) often produces greater symptomatic relief than slow maintenance infusion.

Morning symptoms are common:

Symptoms may worsen in the morning due to overnight fluid shifts and relative hypovolemia.

Some patients benefit from early morning medication dosing before getting out of bed.

Heat worsens symptoms:

Hot environments and showers may provoke vasodilation and orthostatic symptoms.

Patients may require cooler environments and pacing strategies.

Raynaud's vs blood pooling:

Dependent mottled discoloration that improves when limbs are elevated may represent blood pooling rather than true Raynaud's phenomenon.

Compression matters:

Abdominal compression often provides greater benefit than leg-only compression garments.

Medication Quick Reference

Medications may target several physiologic mechanisms involved in dysautonomia.

Common categories include:

• volume expansion agents

• vasoconstrictors

• heart rate control medications

• autonomic modulators

• neuropathic pain agents

• stimulants for fatigue and cognitive dysfunction

Medication selection should be individualized based on symptom patterns, heart rate. and blood pressure responses.

IV Fluids and Volume Expansion

Intravenous fluids may provide temporary symptomatic relief for some patients with severe orthostatic intolerance.

Rapid administration of isotonic fluids often produces greater symptomatic improvement than slow infusion.

Typical protocols include:

500–1000 mL of normal saline administered over approximately one hour.

Rapid bolus administration appears to produce greater symptomatic improvement than slow continuous infusion (for example 125 mL/hour), likely due to more immediate intravascular volume expansion.

Patients frequently report improvement lasting approximately 24–36 hours.

One liter of normal saline contains approximately 9 grams of sodium chloride, equivalent to approximately 154 mEq of sodium.

Special Situations

Certain clinical situations require additional consideration.

Pregnancy

Management should be coordinated with obstetrics or maternal-fetal medicine specialists.

Commonly used medications that may be considered in select cases include beta blockers, pyridostigmine, desmopressin, and intravenous fluids.

Procedures and Surgery

Patients with dysautonomia may experience exaggerated hemodynamic responses during procedures.

Some clinicians recommend administration of 2–3 liters of intravenous fluids prior to minor procedures.

Additional considerations include careful positioning to avoid joint injury in connective tissue disorders and recognition that recovery may be prolonged.

Referral and Red Flags

Possible Neurodegenerative Autonomic Disorders

Although most patients presenting with orthostatic intolerance have non-degenerative dysautonomia such as POTS or neurally mediated hypotension, clinicians should remain alert for features suggestive of **neurodegenerative autonomic disorders,** including:

• Multiple System Atrophy (MSA)

• Pure Autonomic Failure (PAF)

Features that may warrant referral to a neurologist with autonomic expertise include:

• Onset of severe autonomic dysfunction after age 60

• Prominent supine hypertension with orthostatic hypotension (see NOH)

• Progressive neurologic symptoms (parkinsonism, gait changes, cerebellar signs)

• Significant urinary retention or erectile dysfunction early in disease course

• Rapid clinical progression

Neurogenic Orthostatic Hypotension (NOH)

Neurogenic orthostatic hypotension should be considered when orthostatic hypotension occurs with impaired autonomic reflexes and is accompanied by significant supine hypertension, **particularly in older patients or those with neurologic features such as parkinsonism, gait instability, or urinary retention.**

When these features are present, referral to neurology or an autonomic specialist is recommended.

Clinical Tools

These quick-reference tools summarize practical management strategies for clinicians caring for patients with POTS and related dysautonomias.

POTS Clinical Algorithm

Step 1 – Identify Orthostatic Pattern

Consider dysautonomia when patients report:

• Orthostatic lightheadedness

• Palpitations or tachycardia when upright

• Fatigue or exercise intolerance

• Brain fog or cognitive slowing

• Nausea or early satiety

• Heat intolerance

• Blood pooling in the legs or hands

• Symptoms that improve when lying down

If orthostatic intolerance is suspected, proceed with structured evaluation.

Step 2 – Confirm Orthostatic Physiology

Preferred methods:

• Tilt Table Test (if available)

• 10-Minute Stand Test in clinic

Diagnostic clues may include:

• HR increase ≥30 bpm within 10 minutes of standing (≥40 bpm adolescents)

• Orthostatic symptoms reproduced during standing

• Low or narrow pulse pressure

• Orthostatic hypotension or mixed responses

Clinical context remains essential. Many patients present with mixed dysautonomia patterns.

Step 3 – Exclude Alternative Causes

Consider screening for:

• Anemia

• Thyroid dysfunction

• Electrolyte abnormalities

• Endocrine disorders

• Cardiac arrhythmias

• Medication effects

Red flags requiring additional evaluation include:

• New onset symptoms after age 65

• Significant supine hypertension with orthostatic hypotension

• Progressive neurologic symptoms

• Unexplained syncope

Step 4 – Begin Foundational Management

Initial management typically includes:

Volume expansion:

• Increase oral fluid intake

• Increase sodium intake

• Consider oral rehydration solutions

Physical countermeasures:

• Compression garments

• Physical conditioning beginning with recumbent exercise

• Activity pacing

Step 5 – Target Dominant Symptoms

Medication selection should be guided by the patient's primary symptom burden.

Examples include:

• Tachycardia → beta blockers or ivabradine

• Hypotension → midodrine or droxidopa

• Fatigue/brain fog → stimulants, LDN, or volume optimization

• MCAS-type symptoms → antihistamines or cromolyn

• Sleep dysregulation → clonidine or guanfacine

Most patients require layered treatment approaches rather than a single medication.

Step 6 – Reassess and Adjust

Follow-up should evaluate:

• Symptom response

• Blood pressure tolerance

• Medication interactions

• Functional improvement

Treatment should be adjusted gradually with attention to patient tolerance.

Symptom-Guided Medication Table

Symptom Pattern	Possible Medication Options	Clinical Notes
Tachycardia / palpitations	Beta blockers, Ivabradine	Often first-line for HR control
Orthostatic hypotension	Midodrine, Droxidopa	Vasoconstrictors improve upright BP
Fatigue / brain fog	LDN, stimulants, modafinil	Use cautiously in hyperadrenergic patients
Poor sleep / "tired but wired"	Clonidine, Guanfacine	May reduce nighttime sympathetic activation
MCAS-type symptoms	H1 blockers, H2 blockers, Cromolyn	Consider if flushing, itching, hives, rashes, GI symptoms
Volume depletion	Fludrocortisone, Desmopressin	Monitor serum potassium and serum sodium
GI dysmotility / constipation	Mestinon	May improve autonomic signaling.

Many medications may address multiple symptoms simultaneously, and dosing often requires careful titration.

Pocket Reference: Dysautonomia Quick Guide

Recognize the Pattern

Think dysautonomia when patients report:

• Symptoms worsen upright

• Symptoms improve lying down

• Unexplained tachycardia

• Fatigue disproportionate to activity

• Blood pooling or temperature dysregulation

Simple Clinical Tests

• Orthostatic vitals

• 10-minute stand test

• Morning blood pressure patterns

Initial Treatment Priorities

1. Fluids and sodium

Many patients benefit from increased sodium intake and aggressive hydration.

2. Compression

Compression garments may improve venous return and reduce pooling.

3. Medication when indicated

Target the patient's dominant symptom cluster rather than treating a diagnosis label alone.

Clinical Pearls for Dysautonomia

These practical observations may help clinicians recognize and manage dysautonomia in busy clinical settings.

1. The "P" in POTS is Postural

If symptoms improve rapidly when the patient lies down, orthostatic dysautonomia should be considered.

Persistent dizziness even while lying down may suggest vestibular or neurologic causes instead.

2. Patients Are Often Not "Dehydrated"

Many patients with POTS have normal laboratory markers of hydration.

However, they may be chronically intravascularly depleted, meaning plasma volume is insufficient for upright circulation despite adequate total body water.

Increasing sodium intake and plasma volume may significantly improve symptoms.

3. Volume Expansion Makes Medications Work Better

Medications such as:

• Midodrine

• Droxidopa

• Fludrocortisone

• Desmopressin

Medications often work more effectively when plasma volume is optimized through sodium and fluid intake.

4. Morning Symptoms Are Often Worse

Overnight fluid shifts and nocturnal diuresis can worsen morning orthostatic intolerance.

Some patients benefit from:

• Sodium intake before bed

• Desmopressin in selected cases

• Taking midodrine upon waking before getting out of bed

5. Heat Intolerance Is Common

Heat causes peripheral vasodilation, which worsens blood pooling and reduces cerebral perfusion.

Patients frequently report:

• fatigue after showers

• post-shower lightheadedness

• severe symptoms in hot environments

Cooling strategies may significantly improve function.

6. Symptoms Often Flare After Stressors

POTS and related dysautonomias frequently develop or worsen after:

• viral illness

• surgery

• concussion or trauma

• pregnancy

• significant psychological stress

Symptom onset may occur weeks to months after the triggering event.

7. Mixed Dysautonomia Patterns Are Common

Many patients do not fit neatly into one subtype.

Features of:

• hypovolemic

• neuropathic

• hyperadrenergic

There may be patterns that often overlap in the same patient.

Treatment may require addressing multiple physiologic mechanisms.

8. Blood Pooling Can Mimic Raynaud's

Dependent extremities may develop:

• reddish

• bluish

• mottled discoloration

Unlike Raynaud's, these changes often occur with warmth, standing, or heat exposure rather than cold.

9. Chest Pain May Occur Despite Normal Cardiac Testing

Patients may report chest pain with:

• normal ECG

• normal cardiac enzymes

• normal imaging

This may reflect vascular spasm or impaired autonomic regulation rather than structural heart disease.

10. Listen to the Pattern

Patients with dysautonomia often present with multiple seemingly unrelated symptoms.

Recognizing the pattern of orthostatic intolerance may prevent years of fragmented care and unnecessary testing.

Quick Dysautonomia Screening Checklist

Consider dysautonomia when a patient reports multiple symptoms that worsen upright and improve when lying down.

Common features include:

• lightheadedness or dizziness when standing

• rapid heart rate or palpitations

• fatigue or exercise intolerance

• brain fog or difficulty concentrating

• nausea, early satiety, or abdominal discomfort

• heat intolerance or temperature dysregulation

• blood pooling or mottled discoloration of the legs

• frequent need to sit or lean when standing

Additional clues that often appear in dysautonomia patients:

• symptoms began after viral illness, surgery, concussion, or another physiologic stressor

• symptoms fluctuate day-to-day or worsen with dehydration, heat, or illness

• normal routine testing despite significant symptoms

• improvement when lying down or elevating the legs

If several of these features are present, evaluation for orthostatic intolerance or dysautonomia should be considered.

Rapid Clinical Question

A useful screening question for patients:

> "Do your symptoms improve when you lie down?"

A yes answer strongly suggests an orthostatic component.

Important Reminder

Many patients do not present with a single classic syndrome.

Mixed presentations involving hypovolemia, vascular dysregulation, and autonomic instability are common.

Clinical pattern recognition is often more informative than isolated test results.

Sodium Sources for Management

Source	Approximate Sodium Content	Notes
Normal Saline (1 L)	~154 mEq sodium (~3.5 g elemental sodium)	Rapid bolus may provide temporary symptom relief Effects may last 24–36 hours in some patients
Lactated Ringer's (1 L)	~130 mEq sodium (~3 g elemental sodium)	Slightly lower sodium than saline
Trioral oral rehydration packet	~1695 mg sodium per packet	|Mixed with 1 liter water
Typical electrolyte drinks	~200–500 mg sodium per serving	Often lower sodium than needed for dysautonomia
Salt tablets (1 g NaCl)	~390 mg elemental sodium	May be used to increase sodium intake
High sodium diet targets	Often 3–10 g elemental sodium daily	Individualized based on patient tolerance

Practical Reminder

Patients often require more sodium than classical sports/electrolyte drinks provide.

Clinicians should review actual sodium content when recommending hydration strategies.

Clinical Context

Many dysautonomia patients are described as "dehydrated" based on symptoms despite having normal laboratory markers.

In many cases the issue is relative intravascular depletion rather than total body dehydration.

Increasing sodium intake may help expand plasma volume and improve orthostatic tolerance.